THE
NOOTROPICS
GUIDE

GEORGE MIHALACHE

DEDICATION

For each person trying to improve, so today may
you will be better than yesterday!

CONTENTS

ACKNOWLEDGMENTS

I choose to not be limited by my own limits. There are many way to dare into the unknown, and using nootropics is only one of them. But we are improving and enhancing our possibilities with each step in the upward direction. I thank you all the people who think in the same way like me.

NOOTROPICS - INTRODUCTION

Nootropics, also known as smart drugs or cognitive enhancers, are drugs, supplements or other substances that may improve cognitive function (executive functions, memory, creativity, motivation). The word nootropic was coined in 1972 by a Romanian chemist and psychologist, Corneliu Giurgea, derivate from the greek words nous (mind) and trepetin (bending). The most used nootropic is the well-known caffeine.

ACETIL-L-CARNITINE

Acetil-L-Carnitine is a precursor for the aminoacid L-Carnitine.

Benefits:

- helps the body to produce energy;
- it is important for heart and brain function, muscle movement and other body processes;
- improves memory problems related to old

age and memory loss;
- improves feelings of mental and physical tiredness in older people;
- helps symptoms related to declining male hormones (taken for six months improves sexual dysfunction, depression and fatigue in a similar way with the testosterone hormone);
- good for alcohol withdrawal (using IV for 10 days, or orally for 80 days), reducing the withdrawal symptoms;
- slows the rate of progression of Alzheimer's disease;
- improves memory, some of the mental function and behavior;
- poor blood flow to the brain - one single IV dose seems to produce short term improvements;
- improve memory in case of alcoholism;
- reduces blood levels of ammonia (improving liver function and mental function in people with poor brain function due to liver failure);
- treating male infertility and Peyronie's disease (reduces pain and slows the condition becoming worse)

- seems to increase survival and improve physical condition in ALS, especially if it is combined with Riluzole;
- may help in neuropathy (nerve pain), fibromyalgia, fragile x-syndrome, multiple sclerosis, schizophrenia, sciatica (when combined with alpha lipoic acid);
- it is a mitochondrial boosting supplement, helps your muscle mitochondria by burning fat, increase endurance, faster recovery. Fat uses carnitine to be carried to the mitochondria;
- when exercising, increase strength, burns more fat, boosts testosterone, speeds recovery, better insulin sensitivity, builds muscle, reduces muscle fatigue;
- better overall cognitive ability, even reversing dementia in some cases;
- increases glutathione's levels;
- improves focus and attention, helps in ADHD.

Side effects:

- do not use if pregnant or breastfeeding;
- do not use in neuropathy caused by taxanes (chemotherapy drugs);

- might interfere with thyroid, do not use if your thyroid is under-active;
- do not use if you have seizures.

Dosage:
- 1-4 g per day improves mood and decrease depression symptoms for some people;
- reduces nerve pain (neuropathy) caused by diabetes (1000 mg 2-3 times per day);
- for healthy adults, 1-3 g per day for 3-12 months.

BACOPA MONNIERI

Bacopa, also known as Herb of Grace, Bacopa Monnieri, Brahmi, Indian Pennywort, Jalanimba, was used in Ayurveda for long time. (Do not confuse it with Gotu Kola, also called sometimes Brahmi.)

Benefits:

- it is commonly used to improve ADHD symptoms, Alzheimer's disease, anxiety;

- protects brain cells from chemicals involved in Alzheimer's disease;
- improves memory and hand-eye coordination (more efficient for children);
- might prevent some kind of seizures, if you got epilepsy;
- may be useful in case of asthma, back ache, joint pain, sexual problems;
- slows the heartbeat.

Side effects:

- it is safe orally, short term (up to 12 weeks);
- do not use it if pregnant or breast feeding;
- slows down the heart beat;
- do not use it if you have ulcers or lung conditions (increase the secretion of the fluid);
- careful in case of thyroid disorders (might increase thyroid hormone).

Dosage:

- no appropriate dose established, depends of age, health, thyroid activity and other conditions.

COENZYME Q10

The antioxidant coenzyme Q10 is decreasing with age and it is associated with several diseases and genetic disorders when it is at low levels, but it is not the cause. Our cells use Q10 to turn carbs into ATP (which is essential for healthy metabolism, bones, neurological and muscular functions. Also works as an antioxidant, if it is combined with vitamins E, C and Selenium to prevent free radical damage to our cells.

Benefits:

- helps in the treatment of high blood pressure and heart failure;
- enhances the immune system abilities;
- improves symptoms of chronic fatigue;
- reduces high cholesterol levels in blood;
- assists in cancer treatment (by protecting the organs from the chemotherapy drugs side effects);
- treatment of gum disease;
- helps in Alzheimer's and Parkinson disease;
- increase sperm count and motility;
- prevents and treats migraine.

Side effects:

- may interact with other medications (taken for heart failure, diabetes, liver or kidney);
- very rare cases of nausea or heartburn.

Dosage:

- 30-200 mg per day.

CREATINE MONOHYDRATE

Creatine Monohydrate is a natural supplement to boost athletic performance, by helping the muscle to produce more energy, increasing the muscle phosphocreatine stores (phosphocreatine is a precursor of ATP, so you will produce more ATP to continuously perform at maximum intensity).

Benefits:

- supports muscles development by boosting the formation of the proteins that create new muscle fibers;

- increase muscle mass, increase the water content of the muscles;
- reduces the myostatin (molecule responsible for reducing muscle growth), helping the muscle to build faster;
- improves high intensity exercises, improving factors such as strength, ballistic power, sprint ability, endurance, recovery, fatigue resistance, brain performance;
- most effective muscle building supplement, increasing both short term and long term muscle mass;
- helps in Parkinson disease preventing the dopamine decrease and improving muscle strength and function;
- few other neurological diseases had symptoms such as phosphocreatine reduction in the brain (Alzheimer's, ischemic stroke, epilepsy, brain or spinal cord injuries - even ALS, as it is improving muscle function, reduce muscle loss and extends survival by 17%);
- lowers blood sugar level and helps in diabetes;
- useful for the brain, increases the phosphocreatine reserves helping to create more ATP, needed for difficult, complex tasks;

• increase dopamine levels and mitochondrial function (20-50% improvement in memory and recall ability)
• reduces age related memory loss and protects against neurological diseases;
• reduces fatigue and tiredness.

Side effects:

• drink plenty of extra water when used and avoid dehydration (it is bad for your kidneys and creatine increases the risk);
• long term use is not recommended in bipolar disorder;
• caffeine and creatine together can make Parkinson worse (avoid caffeine if it is the case);
• because of the water retention, do not use it if you have kidney problems.

Dosage:

• it is safe and easy to use;
• got a loading phase (20g per day for 4-7 days, then maintenance 1-10 g per day).

GINKGO BILOBA

Ginkgo Biloba, also known as Maidenhair, is a living fossil, used in traditional Chinese medicine (seeds and leaves). Today we use Ginkgo extract, made from the leaves.

Benefits:

- contains high levels of flavonoids and terpenoids (both of them powerful antioxidants fighting the damaging effects of the free radicals - anti-ageing;
- has the ability to reduce inflammation caused by various conditions;
- can increase the blood flow dilating the blood vessels, helps with poor circulation;
- might help in some cases of Alzheimer's and other forms of dementia, especially if it is used alongside the conventional treatment;
- may improve mental performance in healthy people;
- may help to treat anxiety and had the potential to treat depression;
- may be effective for some types of headaches;

- may help with respiratory diseases due to its anti-inflammatory effects;
- may reduce PMS symptoms;
- may improve symptoms of sexual dysfunction.

Side effects:

- do not use in case of allergy to alkyl phenols;
- can increase the risk of bleeding (do not mix with warfarin, aspirin, Prozac, Zoloft, ibuprofen and Tylenol);
- to some people can induce dizziness, headaches, nausea.

Dosage:

- 120-140 mg divined into several doses during the day (effects can be noticed after at least six weeks).

GINSENG

We have 2 different kind of Ginseng - The Asian one (Panax Ginseng) and the American one

(Panax Quinquefolius). Both of them are supposed to boost energy, lower blood sugar, and lower cholesterol levels, reduce stress, promote relaxation, and help in diabetes treatment and with sexual dysfunction for men. The chemical components found in Ginseng, ginsenosides, are responsible for the clinical effect of the herb.

Benefits:

- may help stimulate physical and mental activity in people who feel tired (good results in helping cancer patients undergoing treatment with fatigue);
- may improve thinking process and cognition;
- the ginsenosides have anti-inflammatory effects;
- can treat erectile dysfunction;
- there is a link between ginseng and the treatment and prevention of influenza and respiratory syncytial virus;
- may help lower blood sugar and help treat diabetes as it is improving the insulin resistance;

- increase the general well-being of the one using it.

Side effects:

- it is safe to consume but may give headaches, sleep problems, edema, diarrhea, dry mouth and can make changes in the blood pressure and the blood sugar level;
- do not mix with antidepressants (MAOIs class), heart medication, blood thinners (warfarin, aspirin);
- may increase the effect of caffeine;
- can cancel the effect of the painkillers like morphine.

Dosage:

- the recommended dose is 200-400 mg per day, but it is bio-active from a dose of 40 mg per day.

GOTU KOLA

Gotu Kola, also known as Centella Asiatica or Asian pennywort, is native to Asian wetlands and it is used as a medicinal herb in Ayurveda and Chinese traditional medicine, but also in cooking too.

Benefits:

- contains certain chemicals that decrease inflammation and blood pressure in veins;
- seems to increase collagen production, helping wound healing;
- orally taken for 4-8 weeks seems to improve circulation and reduce swelling in the legs if you got poor circulation
- taking it for 12 months in atherosclerosis stabilize the fatty deposit plaques in the blood vessels making it less likely to break leading to heart attack or stroke;
- prevents blood clots during long flights (more than 3 hours);
- improve mental function;
- might help reduce symptoms of psoriasis, and used as a cream prevents scarring;

- helps bladder wounds healing after parasitic infection called schistomiasis;
- as a cream can heal stretch marks associated with pregnancy;
- useful for fatigue, anxiety, bacterial and viral infections like common cold, flu, tonsillitis, sunstroke, U.T.I., hepatitis, jaundice, diarrhea, indigestion;
- refreshing energy
- used for aging skin, tones and tighten the skin due to collagen production, increase the blood flow, helping in cellulitis;
- strengthen the hair follicles and nourishes the scalp (strengthens the blood vessels in the scalp area and leads to hair regrowth);
- rejuvenative nervine, bringing balance to the nervous system;
- sharpens the mind, increase memory learning and cognition;
- repair and reverse the damage to the brain cells, preventing degenerative brain diseases like Alzheimer's disease;
- boosts acetylcholine production, decreasing the symptoms in ADHD and ADD;
- increases the dendrite and axon growth;
- rich in triterpene saponozides (a Japanese research shows that some of them can stop

the growth of the cancer cells);
- neurogenesis and neuroprotection.

Side effects:

- safe for pregnant women as a cream, not enough data when used orally if the woman is pregnant or breastfeeding;
- cause sleepiness if used in combination with other drugs after surgery (interacting with sedatives, CNS depressants);
- moderate interaction with hepatotoxic drugs (Tylenol, tegretol, simvastatin).

Dosage:

- safe dose for blood circulation 60-180 mg per day;
- recommended 50-250 mg three times per day;
- as a nootropic 3 x 200 mg per day.

LIPOSOMAL GLUTATHIONE (GSH)

The Liposomal Gluthatione is the most powerful antioxidant, combating the effects of physical and emotional stress, pathogens, toxins, free radicals, herbicides, smoking side effects and even ageing). Higher blood and intra-cellular levels of GSH can prevent the oxidization of the cellular membrane, protecting the body from the effects of free radicals. Helps activate vitamin E and C. The liposomal glutathione is protected by the stomach acidity, being assimilated as liposomes and it is 100% bioavailable. GSH is a tripeptide made from cysteine, glutamine and glycine. The highest concentration is found stored in liver.

Benefits:

- plays a key role in detoxifying the body;
- GGT, which can breakdown in GSH, can be taken intravenous, intramuscular, oral or inhaled;
- cellular GSH levels are a good predictor of life expectancy;
- prevents different body systems from deterioration and disease;
- reduces the risk of cancer, Parkinson,

Huntington and Alzheimer's disease;
- prevents glaucoma and cataract;
- fight oxidative stress in the body;
- may control inflammation;
- drops with age, especially during the menopause, increasing the blood levels will prevent age related cognitive decline;
- may prevent depression;
- may limit neurodegeneration;
- may help with infections;
- protects the intestinal mucosa, heals the gut;
- autistic children have 20-40% lower levels of GSH;
- regulation of life, proliferation and death of the cancer cells;
- helps in ADHD;
- prevents heart diseases caused by oxidative stress in the heart tissue;
- may treat diabetes complication in diabetes type 2;
- may prevent kidney and liver disease and kidney failure caused by oxidative stress;
- may decrease the development of addictive behaviors and eating disorders;
- reduces the consequences of alcohol and drugs use;

- controls the activation of cells death pathway;
- may help in asthma and COPD, and in sleep apnea, as they are characterized by lower GSH levels;
- may treat acne, rheumatoid arthritis;
- encourage a healthy pregnancy;
- helps in AIDS and cystic fibrosis;
- it is a skin lightening agent.

Side effects:

- if inhaled can lead to breathing difficulty, do not use it if you have asthma;
- taste bad, liposomal form is recommended, if you are poor, start slow and increase gradually;
- 1 in 8 subjects can experiment increased flatulence, diarrhea or chest tightness.

Dosage:

- not more than 600 mg per day, ideally inhaled
- it is not very effective oral taken, but it is good as liposomal, sublingual or orobucal (lozenges) and increase the vitamin C absorption;
- can be combined with cysteine, selenium, alpha-lipoic acid (ALA) and methionine.

NICOTINAMIDE RIBOSIDE

Nicotinamide Riboside is a precursor to NAD+ (nicotinamide adenine nucleotide). It is a nucleoside made out of niacinamide and ribose. It is a form of the vitamin B3.

Benefits:

- it is an anti-aging and help support healthy circadian rhythm;
- generate energy in mitochondrial dense tissues like muscle, brain and liver;
- protects the mitochondria, improve the mitochondria function and health;
- increase the amplitude of your circadian rhythm (fluctuation of cellular production that coordinate the day-night cycle - poor circadian rhythm lead to lower levels of NAP-MT enzyme, resulting in lower NAD+ levels);
- NAD+ activates the sirtuins * (antiaging enzymes), PARPs (repairs the damaged cells - anticancer effect) and CD38 receptor in the immune system (involved in the glucose-induced insulin secretion-reducing

the diabetic symptoms);
- supports tissues that heavily relies on mitochondria for energy (nervous system, heart, liver, muscle);
- rapidly restore muscle mass;
- protects the brain (protects nerve cells by activating Sirt3(r) and PGC1a(r) pathways);
- protects the liver (stopping the fat accumulation, lowering oxidative stress, preventing inflammation and improving insulin sensitivity);
- increase the metabolism and energy use, increase the level of enzymes involved in burning fat;
- helps reprogram dysfunctional cells, increasing longevity.

Side effects:

- worsen the physical performance (lowest adverse effects - 1000 mg/day, no adverse effect -300 mg/day)

Dosage:

- at 1000 mg, effects start to feel after 6 pills, if you take 2 per day.

* Sirtuins are a family of proteins that act predominantly as NAD-dependent deacetylases. We got Sirt3, Sirt4 and Sirt5 - localized exclusively in mitochondria. Sirtuins are influencing ageing, transcription (DNA copy), apoptosis (programmed cellular death), inflammation, stress resistance, as well as energy efficiency and alertness. During low calorie situations, the sirtuins will control the circadian clock and the mitochondrial biogenesis.

OMEGA 3

Omega 3 - or as it is called n-3 polyunsaturated fatty acids (PUFA), are the following: linolenic acid, EPA and DHA, also known as fish oil fatty acids. Their properties are different than n-6 polyunsaturated fatty acids (PUFA) and monounsaturated fatty acids (MUFA). Omega 3 fatty acids are believed to lower blood triglyceride levels, reducing V - LDL in liver and stimulating V-LDL metabolism in muscle and tissue. A bit of history: when the Inuit population was checked, they got a low occurrence of cardio-vascular diseases (CVD). Their diet is abundant in fatty fish and fish oil, so we reach the conclusion that this provides protection against different CVD. The following research discovered that this diet can provide a 0% to 40% reduction of CVD risk (again, the individual factor is prevalent) and decrease the risk of fatal CVD, but no effect was noted on heart dysfunctions (fibrillation and arrhythmia). In conclusion: we do not have enough data to gather strong evidence, but today we have excellent treatment options, so if you survive the first hearth attack, chances are that the second will never happen (we got statins, blood thinners, beta blockers, blood pressure lowering medicine). N-3 PUFA, or Omega 3 as they are widely known, are effective for high triglycerides, likely effective for heart disease and possible effective for blood pressure, rheumatoid arthritis and weight loss. They have potent anti-inflammatory actions. So, not only does our body need Omega 3 fatty acids to function, but them also delivering some important benefits. It is good to be delivered by food, not by supplements. Sources of Omega 3 are: fish (wild salmon, tuna, sardines, and trout), walnuts, flaxseed, canola oil, soybean oil. The fish is rich in Omega 3 but can also have higher levels of contaminants (mercury, PCB and other powerful toxins). Children and pregnant women should avoid fatty fish. All the foods containing Omega 3 are rich in calories, so moderation is recommended. Algae can be a good replacement if you do not eat fish.

Benefits:

- lower the risk of heart disease by lowering elevated triglycerides blood levels;
- can curb stiffness and joint pain, can boost the effectiveness of the anti-inflammatory drugs;
- lower the depression risk, boosting the antidepressant effects, may help with the depressive symptoms of the bipolar disorder;
- it is very important in the infant visual and neurological development;
- helps in asthma, lowering the inflammation and improving the lung function, cutting the amount of medication needed to control the condition;
- reduces the symptoms of ADHD, but should not be used as primary treatment;
- protection against Alzheimer's disease and

dementia, positive effects on memory loss due to ageing.

Side effects:

- Omega 3 supplements can make bleeding more likely, if you have a bleeding condition and use medication like warfarin, you should ask your doctor before taking Omega 3 supplements.

PTEROSTILBENE

Pterostilbene is a derivative of Resveratrol, but is better absorbed following oral ingestion and more potent as an antioxidant and anticancer molecule. It is ideal to combine with Nicotinamide Riboside as supplement.

Benefits:

- anti-inflammatory, antioxidant, anti-ageing;
- increasing longevity;
- good for anxiety, neuroinflammation, blood pressure, cholesterol, diabetes, joint inflammation.

Side effects:

- up to 250 mg (2 doses of 125 mg per day) with no side effects.

Dosage:

- low doses - beneficial for memory and cognition;
- higher doses (250-500 mg) - beneficial for reducing cholesterol and glucose

RESVERATROL

Resveratrol is a stilbenoid, a type of natural phenol, and a phytoalexin produced by several plants in response to injury or if the plant is under attack by pathogens.

Benefits:

- acting as antioxidant, protecting the body against risks of cancer and heart disease;
- limits the spread of cancer cells and it is killing them;

- reduce inflammation;
- lover LDL and prevents clots to form (avoiding heart attack);
- may ease joint pain;
- may protect nerve cells from damage and fight the plaque build-up leading to Alzheimer's;
- helps in diabetes preventing insulin resistance;
- sirtuins can be activated by resveratrol.

Side effects:

- might interact with blood thinners like warfarin, aspirin and ibuprofen;
- raise the chance of bleeding.

Dosage:

- in the research group was used 2000 mg, but the commercial ones contain only 250-500 mg.

RHODIOLA ROSEA

Rhodiola Rosea, also known as golden root, arctic root or rose root, is the root of an adaptogenic plant.

Benefits:

- it is an adaptogenic (helps your body to adapt to stress when consumed) decreasing stress and improving the symptoms of burnout;
- alleviate and fight fatigue;
- reduces the symptoms of depression, by balancing the brain neurotransmitters. As a fun fact, compared with Zoloft (Sertraline) is slightly less effective, but produces fewer side effects and it is better tolerated by the body.
- improves brain function (reduces mental fatigue, improved sleep patterns, increased motivation);
- can improve exercise performance (endurance);
- may help control diabetes symptoms (can lower blood sugar by increasing the number of glucose transporters in the blood);
- may be useful in the treatment of some types of cancer.

Side effects:

- uncommon and mild allergy;
- irritability, insomnia, agitation, activation.

Dosage:

- on empty stomach, 400-600 mg in a single dose. They need to have the standardized 3% rosavins and 1% salidrosides.

Notes:

Notes:

Notes:

ABOUT THE AUTHOR

Got my first company at 16, more than 20 years ago. Just a market stall, but still paid all my university expenses. Accountant for 10 years, then, one day i felt enough is enough, and i left everything. Changed countries, start working in healthcare, 6 years from now, advanced from NVQ 1 to 5. Meanwhile i studied yoga for more than 20 years, learn few languages, studied finances and economy trends, become an angel investor on small scale, start to learn about start-ups, shares, bonds, real estate and other boring stuff. Aiming for Tim Ferris four hour workweek, but I'm not quite there. Training towards a life coach, therapist and motivational speaker career. And all that when I'm still travelling around the world, going to any seminar or movie I'm interested to see, being in a meaningful relation and doing exercises few times a week. In my peak state i am an unstoppable genius, at my lowest I'm just a lazy guy who like to watch Game of Thrones or play League of Legends/Heroes of the Storm/Hearthstone. Average person with amazing skills in a crisis situation. Have driving license, but do not like to drive. Anything except maybe an ATV. Still need to learn Chinese, jump with parachute and play an instrument.

www.ingramcontent.com/pod-product-compliance
Lightning Source LLC
Chambersburg PA
CBHW030544220526
45463CB00007B/2973